Sodium Nutrition Diet Revealed: What You Need To Know About Sodium

"An informational course in nutrition to help you prevent and eliminate disease"

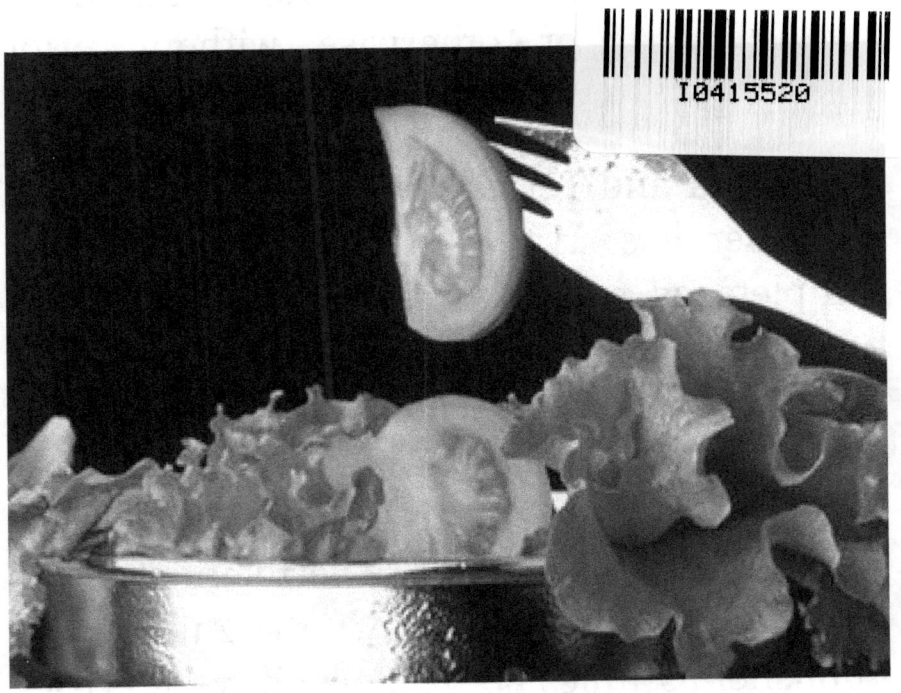

By Rudy S Silva, Natural Nutritionist

Sodium Nutrition Diet Revealed: What You Need To Know About Sodium © 2013 by Rudy S. Silva

ISBN-13: 978-1492969808
ISBN-10: 149296980X

Disclaimer and Terms of Use: The Author and Publisher has strived to be as accurate and complete as possible in the creation of this book, notwithstanding the fact that he does not warrant or represent at any time that the contents within are accurate due to the rapidly changing nature of the Internet. While all attempts have been made to verify information provided in this publication, the Author and Publisher assumes no responsibility for errors, omissions, or contrary interpretation of the subject matter herein. Any perceived slights of specific persons, peoples, or organizations are unintentional. In practical advice books, like anything else in life, there are no guarantees of income made.

Your doctor or health provider should confirm any information given here. This information should not be taken as medical advice, diagnosis, or treatment. This e-book is for information and educational purposes only. If you have any illness or diseases, please see your doctor for treatment and care. Use this information at your own risk.

First Printing, 2013, United States of America

Other Large Print Books from This Author

Head over to Amazon and search for "large print books rudy silva"

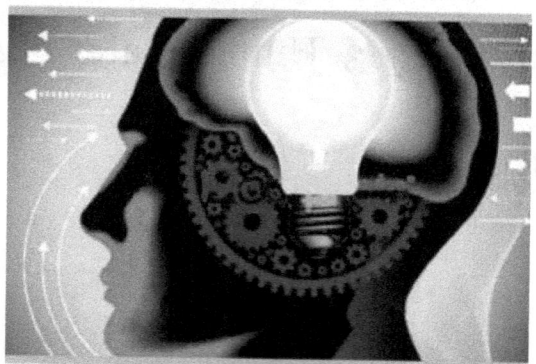

Table of Contents

Chapter 1: Introduction

"Sodium is considered the Youth Element, since in the right proportions in your body, it will keep you young"

Your body has amazing ways that it can prolong your life. Many people and scientist look at the body from a chemical view point, but in fact it is an electrical body. In his book, The Philosopher's Stone, Michiio Kushi recounts how he performed an experiment in his laboratory where he transmuted sodium, $Na+$ into Potassium, $K+$. Having the right sodium in your body can provide transmutation when you need it.

In this Kindle e-book you will discover why you should be concerned about sodium foods and your sodium diet and how this is related to potassium. In the end, it's all about how you can have the best health by minimizing any health problems that can arise from having an imbalance of sodium with respect with other minerals.

Sodium, chloride, and potassium, calcium, magnesium and phosphorus are a few of the critical electrolytes or ions in your body. Sodium is a positive charged electrolyte that resides mostly outside of your body cells.

Sodium stands number one in importance in your body. Ninety percent of the sodium ions, Na+, that exist in the fluids outside of your cells are sodium. It is sodium that attracts fluids and water into the outer cellular area and maintains the balance of these fluids throughout your body.

Sodium is an alkaline mineral that has a positive charge like potassium, that neutralizes acids, whereas potassium helps to drain acids out of the body. The chemical symbol for sodium ions is Na+ and for potassium it is K+. This indicates that Na lacks an electron in its outer orbit and will readily accept an electron so that it can be balanced electrically.

Since Chloride has one extra electron in its outer electron orbit, it can contribute this electron to sodium. The result is that sodium and chloride have an affinity for each other and that is why you see NaCl as a product better known as table salt. You have approximately 3 ounces of sodium in your body.

In the presence of water, NaCl will dissociate into the ions Na+ and Cl-. When you eat foods that contain sodium, your stomach acid will break down your food and in the process release the sodium in the food to form Na+. It is in this form that your body uses Na+ and it is found though out your body eliminating acid. It also serves to create electrical potentials across cell membranes, small littler batteries that help to move nutrients across cell walls.

Many diseases are caused because people lack organic sodium, not table salt, in their diet and are deficient in it in their body liquids. Sodium is called the Youth Element, because if you always have the right amount in your body, you will be limber, pliable, and active. All athletic activities and active hobbies require your body to have plenty of sodium.

Organic Sodium

The difference between organic sodium and inorganic sodium, table salt, is organic sodium is found only in fruits and vegetables. It is alive and has electric magnetic energy and frequencies that your body uses to energizing itself. But inorganic sodium found in table salt and in many other processed foods and is considered dead food. Table salt is not alive and is not the correct sodium that the body needs for good health, but your body will still use it as a substitute when you lack organic salt.

Inorganic Sodium

Salt, sodium chloride, is not a food and is considered inorganic sodium. All inorganic substances are harmful to your body. Salt is crystal found in natural deep in the earth. It's mined and brought up to the surface where it is sorted and purified into various sizes. When it is dissolved by forcing water deep into the earth it is called Brine.

Salt is used in many industries. It is used in thousands of applications from meat packers, food to leather processors. It is used to manufacture glass, soap, and paper. It is used in water, to build roads, refine metals, and make ice cream. It is not a food, but it is used as a seasoning in many foods.

Sodium In Your Body

Like calcium and potassium, sodium has many functions throughout your body and is stored throughout your body, for emergencies. It keeps calcium and magnesium in solution and prevents them from precipitating. It is active in the blood, lymph, lymph nodes, stomach, colon, cells, tissues, and wherever acid is formed in your body.

Sodium maintains the proper extracellular fluid volume, liquid outside cells, since it attracts water. If you have edema, excess water in your body, or high blood pressure, you need to back off on eating salt. When you don't have enough salt, you will lack water in your body. This has a dramatic effect on your blood pressure, since it will cause low blood pressure.

Sodium with the help of potassium and chloride also helps transit impulses in nerve and muscle fibers. All along nerve fibers sodium exists creating an electric voltage across the nerve membranes, so that nerve impulses can travel to the various locations in your body.

Sodium is lost from your body in hot humid weather and when you do hard physical work. Sauna baths, fevers, sweating, passion, extreme excitement also causes sodium loss. Self-abuse and self-hatred also causes loss of sodium. You will also lose sodium when you have an acid body. Sodium is used to neutralize acids and is used up when you have an excess to neutralize.

Sodium also maintains your cell permeability. It moves into your cells and out of your cells as it transports sugars and amino acids into your cells. It is involved in muscle contractions.

Sodium is also found in the blood and there it functions to keep other mineral soluble, so that they do not precipitate out to form deposits. It helps to move carbon dioxide out of your body and is involved in the production of HCL acid in your stomach. It provides a protective layer in your stomach so that HCL does not create ulcers in your stomach lining.

A deficiency in sodium can also result in decreased iron chemical activity. Sodium is needed so that your body can use iron.

Daily Sodium Requirements

You only need around 500 milligrams of sodium per day, but most people who do not watch their salt use get around 4400 to 8800 milligram per day. Since sodium attracts water, eating high levels of sodium each day usually leads to high blood pressure due to extra water in the blood vessels.

Sodium Bicarbonate

Sodium bicarbonate, $NaHCO_3$, or sodium hydrogen carbonate is the common baking soda and many people know this better as Alka-Seltzer. You can use sodium bicarbonate for stomach indigestion for a short time. However, using it long term to alleviate your stomach problems can result in side effects. It is also used to make your blood or urine less acidic.

When sodium bicarbonate is used long term, the bicarbonate part of this chemical, HCO_3, is readily absorbed into the body causing a pH change in your body. This result in a condition called Systemic Alkalosis.

Systemic Alkalosis is a condition where excess bicarbonate ions are in your tissue causing the pH to exceed 7.4. This is the opposite of having an acid body and is a condition where there is an excess of alkaline ions throughout your body. Normally the kidneys will excrete the excess bicarbonate, but there are a few conditions that prevent the kidney from removing the excess bicarbonate, which then leads to Systemic Alkalosis.

One of the effects of alkalosis is an excess of sodium in your body, which comes from the sodium bicarbonate and puts your body's pH out of balance. When you have an excess of sodium in your body, it can lead to a variety of various body conditions – edema, high blood pressure, or cell malfunction.

Some of the side effects of prolong use of sodium bicarbonate, which come from the bicarbonate are:

- severe headache or nausea
- loss of appetite
- irritability or weakness
- frequent urge to urinate
- swelling of legs for feet
- dark or bloody stools
- Blood in urine

Taking sodium bicarbonate pills to relieve an acid body is not recommended. This compound should not be used for medical purposes without direction from a doctor.

Chapter 2: Activities Of Sodium In Your Body

Organic Sodium helps to keep calcium in solution. When your body lacks sodium, calcium will precipitate from solution and create calcium crystals in different parts of your body. When you eat table salt, your body removes calcium from your body and excretes it in your urine.

What you eat and absorb will determine what amount of sodium your body has. The actual sodium requirement of each person differs based on age and size. You need less than 3 grams of sodium daily, but the average American diet provide around 6 gram. It's the kidneys that help to keep excess sodium out of your body, by excreting it in your urine. Other parts of your body will also eliminate sodium – skin, colon, and all liquid discharges.

In his book, Dr. Colgan, Michael, Optimum Sports Nutrition, New York, Advanced Research Press, 1993 say,

"From all the ads for electrolyte replacement drinks for use during and after exercise, you

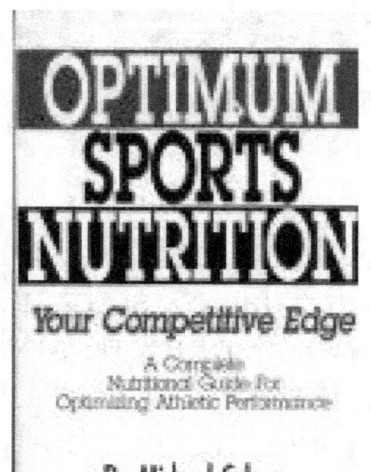

OPTIMUM SPORTS NUTRITION

Your Competitive Edge

A Complete
Nutritional Guide For
Optimizing Athletic Performance

Dr. Michael Colgan

would think that athletes need more sodium. Except for some ultra-distance athletes (Ironman length triathlons, 100-mile running races) that's just promotional flapdoodle. The human body conserves its electrolytes." Dr Colgan says that after exercise you don't need electrolytes or sodium because you lose water during exercise by sweating but your body keeps the electrolytes in your body. You only need to drink water, because now your water to electrolytes is out of balance.

In the beginning of any exercise, you lose some sodium in your sweat, but as you continue your exercise or sport, your body at some point starts to conserve your sodium. The result is that you don't lose much sodium as has been previous thought by many doctors, sports people or people. You don't need those sports drinks that say brings your electrolytes back to normal, when you are working or playing hard.

Sodium and water go together. Sodium attracts water. So if your sodium intake increases and is reflected as an increase sodium in your body, your body will retain more water. The more sodium you have in your body the more water you need to balance this sodium.

When you get thirsty, the posterior pituitary gland will release an anti-diuretic hormone, so that your kidney does not excrete too much water to your bladder. This will help you to maintain the water you have in your body.

When your body sodium decreases, your thirst disappears, the anti-diuretic hormone is suppressed, and the kidney excretes more liquid into your bladder. The result is your body starts to excrete the excess water.

In some cases, you can have an excess of sodium in your body. People who are overweight should decrease their intake of sodium, since sodium attracts water and can add body weight.

Excess sodium has been also associated with a higher risk of cancer, since it upsets the sodium potassium balance. People who eat a diet of high salted foods such as fish, pork, or dried meat upset the sodium potassium balance. The sodium potassium balance is required, since it is these two elements that maintain the right electrical voltage across your body cells. When this voltage is upset, it leads to disease.

What Sodium Does In Your Body

As was mention, one of the key functions of sodium is to maintain your water balance throughout your body and in this process it helps to keep your cells healthy. It is also involved in neutralizing acid molecules that accumulate in your body, from the food you eat, the polluted air you breathe, the negative thoughts you have, or the bad water you drink.

How Sodium Keeps Cells Functioning

Understanding one portion of how your cells work through the use of sodium and potassium is an important step in knowing why you should strive to eat the right sodium foods and to not eat an excess of table salt.

Sodium is found outside and inside of your cells. You have 1000 mg of sodium your body. Fifty percent of that is in your extracellular fluid, outside of your cells, 10% inside of your cells, and 40% in your bones. Typically there are 7% sodium ions inside your cells and 93%

outside your cells. Your size and age determine how much sodium your body needs. What you eat and how you absorb your food will determine how much sodium goes into your body.

Typically, your body needs around 200mg to 500 mg of sodium daily, but it has been found that people intake up to 6000 mg daily. If you have normal functioning kidneys, the amount of sodium maintained in your body is constant. The kidneys will excrete excess sodium from your body. Sodium is also excreted in feces and sweat

In your body sodium and water go together. If you eat too much sodium the water in your body will increase. If you eat less sodium, the amount of water held in the extracellular fluids will decrease.

Your body controls the amount of water you maintain in your body by a diuretic and anti-diuretic hormone that is release to pass more water out your kidney as urine or to not pass water out of your body. When your sodium level increases, your body makes you thirsty so you will drink more water.

Sodium Potassium Pump

Sodium and potassium ions exist outside your cells, extracellular liquid, and inside your cells, intracellular liquid. In the cell, there is around 7% sodium and 92% potassium. Outside the cell there is the opposite, 93% sodium and 8% potassium. These are the percentage that should be maintained for good cellular function. Naturally, sodium tends to diffuse into the cell while potassium tends to diffuse out of the cell.

The sodium-potassium pump is embedded in the cell membrane and opens to move sodium or potassium ions back and forth across from outside to inside or from inside to outside the cells. This is done to keep a certain voltage across the cell membrane. This potential allows sugar or glucose and amino acids to move into the cell using the sodium-potassium pump. As cells use up nutrients brought in, toxic matter is created. This toxic matter is then transported out of the cell using the sodium-potassium pump.

Go to the following link to view sodium pump process.

http://url2it.com/msrc
or
http://url2it.com/msrd

So now you can see the importance of maintain the proper levels of sodium in your body.

Chapter 3: Detrimental Effects of Table Salt To Avoid

Your body does not need table salt. But it does need sodium and chloride, which is found naturally in food. Your body stores sodium and has plenty, if you eat the right kind of food. When you have a poor diet or have a destructive lifestyle, you deplete your sodium.

There are many detrimental effects of eating too much table salt. However, these effects are not related to the sodium you get from the food you eat. This is because the sodium you get from natural food, which has not been cooked, is electrically charged and has energy associated with it. Table salt is a dead food and has no electrical charge associated with it.

Bone Density

When you eat salt, calcium is excreted from your body and this leads to lower bone density. Granted the amount of calcium lost is small, but over time it can be significant. If you drink coffee, then caffeine will cause you to lose a little bit more bone density.

In his book, Kessler, George D.O., P.C. and Kapklein, Colleen, The Bone Density Program, New York, Ballantine Books, 2000, he points out that,

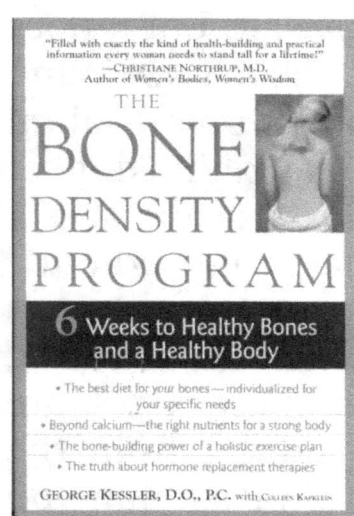

"As with high blood pressure, some people seem to be more sensitive to the effects of salt that others. But the group of sensitive people is large enough that everyone would be wise to use discretion when it comes to salt. Since you don't automatically know whether you are sensitive... Stay within the American Heart Association's guidelines (2,000 mg a day or less) to be safe."

Heart Disease and Cancer

Many studies have been done on how salt contributes to heart disease and cancer. It has been thought that high salt diets contribute to heart diseases.

But in Dr. Watts,L. David, Trace Elements and

Other Essential Nutrients, Texas, 4th Writer;s B-L-O-C-K, 2003, he clarifies studies that point to chlorine as the major contributor to heart and cancer diseases.

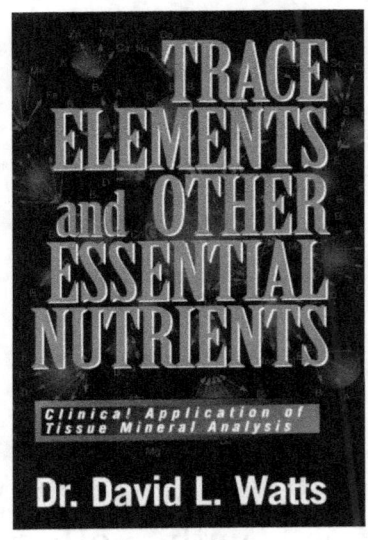

"It now appears that the salt-hypertension link was overly exaggerated. In fact, stringent salt restriction is only necessary for a small segment of the affected population. Only about 10-15 percent may benefit from limiting salt intake. These are a group of individuals with high blood pressure who are classified as 'salt-sensitive.' More recent studies implicate chloride in the development of hypertension rather than sodium alone. Animal studies have shown that high amounts of sodium chloride can induce an elevation in blood pressure."

The actual cause of high blood pressure is not that clear cut, since many people with high blood pressure may have a number of mineral imbalances. Some people are sensitive to sodium and some to chloride and these sensitivities can cause various health issues.

Another factor involved in heart disease is the sodium to potassium ratio. Dr. Julian Whitaker, M.D. points out that most people have a ratio of twice as much sodium as potassium in the body. By changing this ratio, Dr. Whitaker claims you can protect yourself from heart and cancer. To do this you need to watch your salt intake and learn which foods give you more potassium and add them to your diet.

Excess salt has also been known as a stomach cancer threat. This is especially true when the sodium in salt combines with other carcinogens – barbecue smoke, grilled meat, sodium nitrides, or pesticides. Salt irritates the stomach, which increases the disposition of precancerous cell replication and powers chemical carcinogen to do more stomach damage. When your diet is low in fruits and vegetables, the results of a high salt diet are even more damaging.

Kidney Damage

When you eat salt, your body tries to get rid of it. It does this by making you thirsty. If you drink more water, your kidney will cause you to urinate more. This is how your body tries to get rid of the salt you eat.

Of all your body **organs**, your kidneys suffer the most when you eat salt. If you eat more salt than your kidneys can remove, your kidneys breakdown the salt and deposit it in various parts of your body, but mostly in your lower legs. Then your body tries to protect itself from this salt by bringing water to that area. This causes swelling in the legs and feet. This also causes puffy eyelids and bags underneath your eyes.

Fluid Retention and Sodium Restricted diet

In cases where excess sodium has been consumed and where the kidney has not expelled the excess, fluid retention disease starts to appear, if the excess sodium condition continues to exist. Fluid retention diseases are congestive heart failure and edema. Other excess sodium conditions are kidney failure, adrenal disease, and cirrhosis of the liver. Under these conditions, a sodium restricted diet is called for. Using the information in this kindle e-book provides you with a good start in restricting your use of table salt in your diet.

Chapter 4: Sodium Diet Foods You Must Eat

When joints start to get hard and painful to move, they lack nutrients or specific minerals. With arthritis, sodium is lacking, so sodium foods recommended are okra and celery, which are also available in tablets. Goat whey is another good source of sodium and can be purchased on the internet. To get more information on goat whey, just type this word into Google search.

Other fruits and vegetables that are high in sodium should also be eaten. Only fruits that are picked ripe should be eaten. If they are picked green and allowed to become ripe, they will not have as much sodium, since the sun helps to create the sodium in food.

Some people who have symptoms related to sodium deficiencies may recover quickly or may take a long time to benefit from the addition of sodium. It takes up to 3 months to replenish the sodium reserves in your body, when they are low. And this is providing you are eating an excess of fruits and vegetables.

Sodium and the stomach

The stomach is considered a sodium organ, since it stores sodium in its walls to prevent stomach acid from burning a hole in its tissue. As stomach HCl, hydrochloric acid, moves against your stomach walls, sodium neutralizes it, preventing it from damaging your stomach walls.

The sodium you eat first goes to the stomach walls and the excess goes to the joints. So if you have joint problems you most likely have stomach problems also.

Sodium Foods

Raw goat milk and goat whey are foods high in sodium. Black mission figs are also high in sodium.

Here is a broth that you can make to get extra sodium and potassium called Veal Joint Broth as described by Bernard Jensen, Ph.D.

"Use a clean, fresh, uncut veal joint and after washing in cold water, put into a large cooking pot: cover half with water and add the following vegetables and greens cut up finely:

Small stalk of celery

1 ½ cups apple peelings, ½ in thick

2 cups potato peeing, ½ in thick

½ cup chopped parsley

2 beets, grated

1 large parsnip

1 onion

½ cup okra

Simmer all ingredients for 4 or 5 hours: strain off liquid and discard solid ingredients. There should be 1 ½ quarts of liquid. Drink hot or cold and keep refrigerated."

These are the foods high in sodium:

Apples	kale	kelp
Dried apricots	asparagus	barley
Beets	mustard greens	greens
Red cabbage	okra	carrots
Celery	dried pea's	cheeses
Red peppers	coconut	prunes
Collard	sesame	spinach
Dulse	strawberries	egg yolks

Figs	Swiss chard	turnips
Artichokes	lemons	parsley
Lentils	raw milk	beets
Chickpeas	raisins	dates
Sunflower	goat milk	watercress

Every day you should be eating these various vegetables. You want to make sure you eat at least three highly colored vegetables with your lunch and dinner – bright green, red, orange, yellow, purple and so on. The more colors you can include in your meals the healthier you will be.

Minimize Your Use Of Salt

Since you have probably been using salt for a long time, you have become accustom to having a lot of salt in your food. You can use other ways to spice up your food, without using a lot of salt. Here are a few ways to do this.

Use herbs, spices, and culinary herbs

Use lemon or lime juice to flavor your food

Don't use salt in cooking nor have it on your table

Use butter that is salt free. Don't use margarine, since it has trans fatty acids or hydrogenated oils.

Most canned foods or processed foods are high in sodium. Look for those are low sodium or sodium free.

Choose breakfast cereals that are low in sodium

Fresh meat, poultry, fish are low in sodium, avoid the processed meats

Use low sodium soy sauce

Avoid teriyaki sauce and miso sauce, which are very high in sodium

Avoid boiling vegetable with salt added, vegetables will absorb the salt

Use these labels to determine how much sodium is in food you buy per serving. Sodium – Free, contains less than five mg of sodium.

Very low sodium contains less than 34 mg of sodium.

Low – sodium has less than 141 mg of sodium.

Reduced – sodium has 75% of sodium found in normal food.

Salt Replacement

You can completely eliminate the need to use salt in your food preparation or reduce its use to a very low amount. This is done by becoming familiar with spices and culinary herbs. By consistently using herbs and spices you get fantastic good taste and their therapeutically benefits. The best way to use herbs and spices is to read about their use in food and create a blend that you can use over and over.

Here are some spices to consider:

Basil – use in tomato sauces, soups, salads. Place a small amount in your palm then rub both hands to break the tiny flakes and let them fall into your soup.

Cloves – use with pumpkin and squash dishes or to spice up your rice and baked goods dishes.

Garlic – is part of the onion family and it should be used every day and in as many different dishes that you prepare.

Ginger – use it in cooking meat, stir fry, cookies, or cakes.

Paprika – use it to liven up chicken, mashed potatoes or broiled fish.

Red pepper powder – use it in soups, stews, sauces. You can use a variety of different pepper powders. Try the Eagle brand chili powder, which contains more than one type of chili pepper.

Rosemary – used to flavor chicken, turkey, and lamb.

Turmeric – use with curries.

You can get fresh herbs such as basil, dill, parsley, cilantro or mint. Put the dried herbs into your pot early in your cooking. For fresh herbs, wait until near the end of your cooking.

One of the ways to use herbs is to create a blend that you can add to your dishes as you cook them. You can create a blend for different types of dishes that you cook. Through experimenting with different herbs and spice you can make your own blends. Here are a couple of simple blends.

For Italian Dishes – use only the amount you need.

1 tablespoon of dried oregano

1 tablespoon dried basil

1 tablespoon of dried thyme

For **Mexican soups** add and taste

1 tablespoon of dried oregano

1 tablespoon of basil

1 tablespoon of chili powder

1 tablespoon of a variety of chili powders

1/2 tablespoon of cumin

A **general blend** would be like this

1 tablespoon of dried basil

2 teaspoons of celery seed

2 teaspoons of dried savory

1 teaspoon of dried thyme

1 teaspoon of dried marjoram

Sodium bicarbonate

Organic Sodium bicarbonate, $NaHCO_3$, contains sodium, hydrogen, carbon and oxygen and is also known as baking soda. Organic sodium bicarbonate is created in your body and is used when you have mucus congestions in the throat and bronchial areas. When you have these conditions, sodium foods are recommended. Bicarbonate is also called for to reduce gout, diabetic acid, subacid blood, and stomach mucus.

Saliva

Saliva is an alkaline substance, which is used to neutralize acids as they enter your mouth. It is composed of many different alkaline compounds, such as calcium, sodium, and magnesium phosphates, sodium and potassium chlorides, and sodium carbonate.

Sodium is involved in a variety of digestion processes as food goes into your mouth, stomach and small intestine.

Bile

Your bile that comes from your liver into your gallbladder consists of:

- Sodium carbonate
- Sodium phosphate
- Potassium chloride
- Sodium chloride
- Lecithin
- Sodium palmitate
- Sodium stearate
- Cholesterin
- Sodium taurocholate
- Sodium glycocholate
- Water

When your body doesn't have enough sodium, it will take it from your bile in the gallbladder and as sodium is depleted from the bile, cholesterol will precipitate causing gallstones.

Bile is necessary for you to have regular bowel movements, since it stimulates peristaltic colon action. When your liver is not putting out enough bile, you will have constipation.

When you have enough bile your stool will be a light brown.

Hidden Salt

There are many processed foods that contain sodium chloride or inorganic salt. This is the type of salt that creates sickness, when consumed in excess. As you look at the various foods you buy, look at the nutritional label and buy only those foods that have less salt.

In his Bragg Health Series, N.D., PhD, Bragg, G., Paul and Bragg Patricia, N.D., PhD, The Miracle of Fasting, California, Health Science, they recall an incident that shows the deadly power of salt,

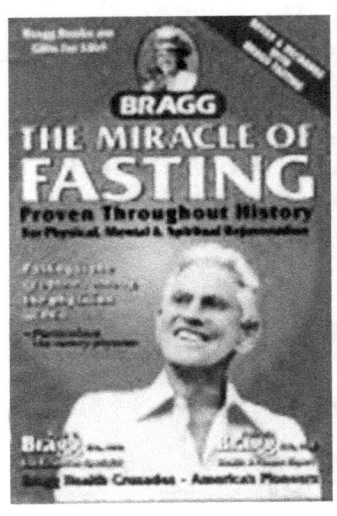

"The most dramatic wrongful death case against salt occurred in a Binghamton, New York hospital, where a number of babies died when salt was inadvertently used in their formula. An overdose of salt can kill a baby quickly. The body needs natural, organic sodium – not table salt, an inorganic chemical. You can obtain natural sodium which Mother Nature provides in organic form in celery, beets, carrots, potatoes, soybeans, turnips sea vegetation, seaweed, kelp, watercress, etc. and many other natural healthy foods. Remember, only organic minerals can be utilized by your body's living cells."

The amount of organic sodium you need per day is up to 500mg. But because there is hidden salt in most processed foods and by your use of table salt, you probable consume from 500 to 6000 mg per day.

Here are a few of the foods with hidden salt to look out for:

- Cured meats – bacon, hot dogs, sliced processed meats, sausages
- Canned soups, canned tuna, prepared pancakes
- TV dinners
- Regular soy sauce
- Tomato sauces
- All packaged foods

Sodium in your drinking water

There is also sodium in the bottled water that you drink. The amount it has is based on the brand. Some bottled water has very little and others have up to 200 mg or more. If you are on a strict sodium diet, then you need to know which bottled water has less sodium.

Most bottle water companies put sodium into their water so that it tastes better. But, some do not and just allow what is in the water to exist. Companies that produce low –salt or no-salt water must list the sodium contain in their bottles.

Water that is labeled Natural Spring Water has sodium but this type of water has the lowest sodium content as compared to other bottled water. If you drink distilled water then there is no sodium in this type of water.

Sodium Compounds Which Attack Your Immune System

Sodium has the ability to form many compound inside and outside your body. Many food suppliers tend to put a variety of sodium compounds in your food to make it taste better or to have a better consistency. These compounds tend to erode cells and tissue creating clumps of deadly free radicals. The result of this is that they use up a lot of your antioxidants that you need elsewhere in your body.

Here is a list of these sodium compounds that you want to avoid. Read the labels on the food you buy and check that the food you buy is free of these compounds.

Salt, sodium chloride – is a destructive compound, which you should eat less of. Get your sodium by eating more sodium foods.

Baking powder – used in various baking products

Baking soda, sodium bicarbonate – used to relieve various stomach issues.

Brine, table salt or water – used in foods to control growth of bacteria and in cleaning fruits and vegetables, in freezing or canning certain foods, and for flavoring corned beef, pickles, sauerkraut, French fries.

Disodium phosphate – used in quick

cooking cereals or processed cheeses.

Monosodium glutamate - comes in many different brands, used in packaged or frozen foods.

Sodium alginate – used in some chocolate milks and ice cream.

Sodium benzoate – used as a preservative in sauces and salad dressings.

Sodium hydroxide – used to soften olives, hominy and some fruits and vegetables.

Sodium propionate – used in pasteurized cheeses, some breads and cakes to inhibit mold.

Sodium sulfite – used to bleach fruits for artificial colors, such as cherries, dried fruit.

Sodium nitrate or sodium nitrite – a dangerous preservative that is used on meat, which is considered carcinogen, cancer forming.

Sodium citrate – a chemical used in food that is harmful to your health.

Sodium dioctyl sulfate, Colace, – used as a lubricant in laxative products and can be habit forming

Chapter 5: Salt Bath Curative Effects

External Use of Salt

Eating sodium is not the only way to get it into your body. It can be used externally as a natural remedy. Salt can be used in many ways to heal and detoxify your body. In combination with water, salt can be applied externally and have a positive effect on your body's pH and health. It is recommended that you use coarse salt or sea salt for your footbath, tub bath, or massage.

The types of salts below can be found by searching on Google. Type in coarse salt and get a variety of sites that sell this type of salt and many others that you can use for your bath.

Here some of the different types of salts you can use:

- Celtic sea salt
- Himalayan Crystal Salt, food grade

- Coarse sea salt
- Dead Sea Bath Salt -
- Epson Salt
- Atlantic Sea Bath Salt

Epson salt is used to create strong perspiration. It is a muscle relaxer and should not be used, if you are not in good health. The Dead Sea salt can help you, if you have had an injury.

What makes these salts great is that you not only have regular salt, $NaCl2$, but they contain many other mineral salts – magnesium and potassium salts.

Not all salts have the same minerals, so you have to check the specifications. Using salts that have a variety of minerals is a great way to get curative effects, when they are used as massage or bath.

Salt Massage Bath

You will want to do a salt massage bath, when you want to stop an oncoming cold, relieve gout pain, restore blood and lymph circulation, overcome sluggishness, and to clean your skin of dirt and dead skin.

This type of massage will improve your mood and reduce your stress as the friction of the salt goes over your skin. It acts as a skin and body stimulant, by increasing blood circulation. If you have a mild case of depression this will help you.

Here's how to do it. Use plain coarse salt, sea salt, or many of the other salts.

Create a slushy salt paste with warm water. You can sit in the tub or shower and pour some salt and water into your hands and create a paste. Apply this paste all over your body from shoulders to feet in a slow circular motion. If you want you can place your feet in hot water as you massage your body. Do the massage only for a few minutes.

After your massage, wash off salt with a gentle shower of slightly warm water and rub your skin with a sponge to remove the salt and stimulate your skin.

If you have any open cuts do not do the salt massage in those areas. Also if you have skin lesions or skin inflammation, do not do the massage.

Complete immersion Salt Bath

Use a salt bath when you need to relax. If you have been sitting in your chair all day and have had a lot anxiety then a salt bath will help you release tension. If you need to clean your skin of dirt or dead skin, a salt bath will help you do this. Women in menopause will benefit for a salt bath.

Here how to do it.

In a tub of warm water put 1 to 2 cups of salt crystals. The more cups you use, the more you will perspire. To simulate sea water you can use 5 pounds of coarse salt and this will act as a mild tonic on your body. You can use water at 65 to 75 F for your bath but stay in the bath for 2 minutes or so. With warmer water you can stay in the bath for up to 15 minutes. Finish your bath with a warm shower and rub your body with a sponge or cloth.

Chapter 6: Sodium Gives You An Alkaline Body

A diet rich in sodium provides the body with the sodium to neutralize acids in your kidney and liver. Sodium works to eliminate acetic, buturic, lactic and other fatty acids, which are derived from starchy foods, lard, margarine, potatoes, oily nuts, and meats. These foods cause the precipitation of sodium and potassium and deplete them, if you continually eaten them.

When sodium is deficient, bad bacteria takes over your digestive tract. In the colon, sodium keeps the environment slightly alkaline to control the bad bacterial.

Sodium Deficiencies

Here are some of the symptoms you will have if you have a deficiency of body sodium:

Gout	cracking joints
Dull complexion	tendons stiff
Restless nerves	fatigue

Mental confusion	drowsiness
Bad breathe	Lack of saliva
Excess mucus	bloating
Constipation	Frontal headache
White coated tongue	

Because fruits and vegetables are naturally grown from soil, they pull minerals out of the ground and can be a great source of minerals like sodium for you. Because of these minerals and other nutrients, fruits and vegetables have amazing curative effects, when they are eaten raw.

If you have acid body, like most people do, this is what is causing your illness. You need to move your acid body into an alkaline condition and sodium and other minerals can help you to do this.

Minerals

Moving your body more toward alkalinity is what will give you the best curative effects of fruits. An alkaline body prevents your body from becoming ill and forming deadly diseases, like all kinds of joint problems, organ degradation, body pain, or even cancer. If you are already sick, then all of the chemicals inside fruits will help to revive you to better health. This is provided that your tissue damage has not gone beyond repair.

The minerals most important in changing and maintaining your body in an alkaline condition are sodium, potassium, chloride, calcium, phosphorus, magnesium, and sulfur.

Now, how your body can become alkaline might become a little confusing at first because of the terms used, but let's break this down into small parts. This process has been discussed in previous chapters, but this explanation gives more details. First we are going to be defining some terms so we can then start talking the same language.

Acid Binding

There are certain minerals that are called acid binding. And these are minerals, as mentioned earlier, are the most important ones in fruits, Sodium, potassium, chloride, calcium, phosphorus, magnesium, because they are acid binding.

What acid binding means is when you eat fruits with these minerals, your cells, after metabolism, create an alkaline ash. This ash will seek out acids in your body and bind with them to neutralize them.

Alkaline Ash

Now, that this alkaline forming ash has tied up an acid it is carried to the kidney where it is expelled as urine.

Different reactions can occur when an acid binding mineral, like say sodium, encounters an acid. Of course acids in the body are toxic, so the body has the priority of getting rid of them fast, since they can damage tissue and cause pain and disease.

Here is another path way of the acid binding mineral process when it combines with an acid.

The Acid Binding Mineral Process

When you eat acid binding food, the blood carries it to the cells where it is oxidized, digested, or metabolized. The result of this digestion is a carbonic acid salt of alkaline minerals, which reacts with body acids and binds with them. In this process, a weak carbonic acid is created. Now, this weak carbonic acid is taken by the blood into the lungs where it is released as carbon dioxide and water.

If not all the acid toxins are captured by acid binding matter, the remaining acids can be neutralized by body stores of alkaline minerals. If you don't have a good store of alkaline minerals, then these acids will remain in your body creating pain and disease.

But if you do have a good store of alkaline minerals, then these minerals will find these acids, capture them and bind with them. Then these acids are routed out through your urine or colon and out of your body.

So you can see the importance of getting a lot of alkaline minerals into your body. Without them, acids which do not get bonded to alkaline minerals would move back into body tissue and continue their body damage.

Alkaline Binding

Now, there are also minerals that become

alkaline binding and these minerals are sulphur, chlorine, iodine, phosphorous, bromine, fluorine, copper, and silicon.

It is these minerals that when digested by a cell will produce an acid salt that will bind with alkaline minerals. These minerals will be excreted through your urine. When alkaline minerals are bonded to an acid salt, the alkaline mineral is removed from your body and your body becomes more acidic, the condition you are trying to avoid.

Although you need to eat both foods that are acid binding or alkaline binding, you want to eat more of the acid binding foods.

Final Comments – The Secrets of Sodium

The difference between organic sodium and inorganic sodium is critical to understand and apply. Organic sodium is only found in natural produce and is available to you when you eat fresh produce. When this produce is stored and sprayed for storage and transport, it loses is potential to provide you with the best sodium and other minerals.

Your body only uses organic sodium because it has electrical energy in the form of ions and frequency. The frequency come from its color and it is this energy that the cells use to provide you with the energy you need to run your body.

Whereas inorganic sodium is in table salt and this is the type of sodium that you find in most grocery store package products. When you eat table salt your body tries to get rid of it. This is why sodium attracts so much water. Through water, your body can eliminate this salt in your urine.

But if you eat too much salt, your kidneys are overwhelmed and can't get rid of all of it. So, it stores this salt in different parts of your body. The result is that you gain weight and develop sickness. Excess body water creates edema. In your cells excess water will appear and now the electrical potential that is between outside and the inside your cell is changed and your cell will not work properly.

Organic sodium is used throughout your body and it first goes to your stomach walls where it is stored to prevent the high stomach acid from burning a hole in your stomach - stomach ulcers. Then it is used to keep your joints from drying out by attracting water to the area needed. Since sodium is part of the Potassium – Sodium Pump, the amount of sodium is closely regulated by your body so that you don't have an excess. Natural food has the proper ratio of potassium and sodium the body needs.

An excess of sodium attracts water and excess water will cause your body cells to function less efficiently. When you are deficient in sodium you will have a variety of symptoms and illnesses that will start to develop. You can maintain adequate supply of sodium in your body, by eating raw fruits and vegetables and goat whey.

Most likely, you will not have an excess of salt, unless you eat a lot of salty meats and use plenty of salt with your meals. Since your body uses sodium to reduce acids in your body, sodium is used up quickly and your sodium reserves can become depleted.

Most people have acid bodies and that's one reason they have various illnesses. What this means is that they are deficient in organic sodium and they are not able to neutralize all of the acid that is created in their body from the acid foods that they eat. Acid foods like meat, potatoes, butter, carbohydrates need to be balanced with alkaline foods like fruits and vegetables. To understand how to change an acid body to an alkaline body check my Kindle e-book called, "Secret Diet And Nutrition (Nutrition Tips: Alkaline Body).

Here is something for you to do to get more natural sodium into your body. Go to the internet and look up goat milk and goat whey. Read about the benefits you can get by using these products. Then the next time you go to a health food store see if they have raw goat milk or goat whey.

They might have raw goat milk depending on what state you live in and mostly likely you can only find goat whey on the internet as "whex." Goat milk is an alkaline food and has a lot of sodium. Even raw cow's milk is alkaline, but when it is pasteurized or homogenized it becomes an acid food.

Appendix A: Choosing The Best Sodium Foods

Here is a more comprehensive list of foods and the amount of sodium they contain. This is based on 3 1/2 cups of the food. This list is to give you an idea of the amount of sodium in both processed foods and fruits and vegetables. You should pick those foods that are more natural and that are not processed, which have the highest sodium value. Those foods with high potassium value are also important.

Meat and Poultry*	Portion	Sodium (mg.)	Potassium (mg.)
Bacon	1 strip (1 oz.)	71	16
Beef			
Corned Beef (canned)	3 slices	803	51
Hamburger	¼ lb.	41	382

Pot Roast (rump)	¼ lb.	43	309
Sirloin Steak	½ lb.	57	545
Chicken (broiler)	31/2 oz.	78	320
Duck	31/2 oz.	82	285
Frankfurter (all beef)	1/8 lb.	550	110

Ham

Fresh	1/4 lb.	37	260
Cured, butt	1/4 lb.	518	239
Cured, shank	1/4 lb.	336	155

Lamb

Shoulder Chop (1)	½ lb.	72	422

Rib			
Chop (2)	½ lb.	68	398
Leg Roast	¼ lb.	41	246

Liver

Beef	31/2 oz.	86	325
Calf	31/2 oz.	131	436

Pork

Loin Chop	6 oz.	52	500
Spareribs (3 or 4)	31/2 oz.	51	360
Sausage (link or bulk)	31/2 oz.	740	140
Turkey	31/2oz.	40	320

Veal

Cutlet	6 oz.	6	448
Loin Chop (1)	1/2 lb.	54	384

Rump Roast	¼ lb.	36	244

Fish

Clams (4 1g.,9 sm.)	31/2 oz.	36	235
Cod	31/2 oz.	70	382
Flounder or Sole	31/2 oz.	56	366

Lobster (1)

Boiled, with 2 tbsp. butter	3/4lb.	210	180

Oysters (5 to 8)

Fresh	31/2 oz.	73	121
Frozen	31/2 oz.	380	210

Salmon (pink, canned)	31/2 oz.	387	361
Sardines (8)			
Canned, in oil)	31/2 oz.	510	560

Shrimp	3 1/2 oz.	140	220
Tuna Canned, in oil	3 1/2 oz.	800	301
Canned, in water	3 1/2 oz.	41	279

Snacks

Candy

Chocolate Creams	1 candy	1	15
Milk Chocolate	1 oz	30	105

Ice Cream

Chocolate	½ pint	75	*
Vanilla	½ pint	82	210

Nuts

Cashews (roasted)	6-8	2	84

Peanuts (roasted)			
Salted	1 tbsp.	69	105
Unsalted	1 tbsp.	trace	111

Olives

Green	2 medium	312	7
Ripe	2 large	150	5
Potato Chips	5 chips	34	88
Pretzels (3 ring)	1 average	87	7

Dairy Products

Butter (salted)	1 pat	99	2
Butter (unsalted)	1 pat	1	2

Cheese

American, cheddar	1 oz.	197	23
American, processed	1 oz.	318	22
Cottage, creamed	31/2 oz.	229	85
Cream (heavy)	1 tbsp.	35	10
Egg	1 large	66	70
Milk (whole)	8 oz.	122	352
Oleomargarine (salted)	1 pat	99	2

Breads Cereals, Etc.

Bread

Rye	1 slice	128	33	56

White (enriched)	1 slice	117	20
Whole Wheat	1 slice	121	63
Corn Flakes	1 cup	165	40
Macaroni (enriched, cooked tender)	1 cup	1	85
Noodles (enriched, cooked)	1 cup	3	70
Oatmeal (cooked)	1 cup	1	130
Rice (white, dry)	¼ cup	3	45
Spaghetti (enriched, cooked tender)	1 cup	2	92

Waffles (enriched)	1 waffle		356	109
Wheat Germ	3 tbsp. 1	232	102

Beverages

Apple Juice	6 oz.	2	187
Beer	8 oz.	8	46
Coca-Cola	6 oz.	2	88
Coffee (brewed)	1 cup	3	149
Cranberry Cocktail	7 oz.	2	20
Ginger Ale	8 oz.	18	1

Orange Juice

Canned	8 oz.	3	500
Fresh	8 oz.	3	496
Prune Juice	6 oz.	4	423
Tea	8 oz.	2	21

Fruits*

Apple	1 medium	1	165
Apricot			
Fresh	2-3	1	281
Canned			
(in syrup)	3 halves	1	234
Dried	17 halves	26	979
Banana	1 6-in.	1	370
Blueberries	1 cup	1	81
Cantaloupe	¼ melon	12	251

Cherries

Fresh	½ cup	2	191
Canned (in syrup)	½ cup	1	124

Dates

Fresh	10 medium	1	648
Dried (pitted)	1 cup (6 oz.)	2	150
Fruit Cocktail	½ cup	5	161
Grapefruit	½ medium	1	135
Grapes	22 grapes	3	158
Orange	1 small	1	200

Peaches

Fresh	1 medium	1	202
Canned 2 halves,	2 tbsp. syrup	2	130

Pears

Fresh	½ pear	2	130
Canned 2 halves,	2 tbsp. syrup	1	84

Pineapple

Fresh	¾ cup	1	146

Canned	1 slice/syrup	1	96

Plums

Fresh	2 medium	2	299
Canned	3 medium, 2 tbsp. syrup	1	142

Prunes

Dried	10 large	8	694
Straw- berries	10 large	1	164
Watermelon	½ cup	1	100

Vegetables*

Artichoke

Base and soft end of leaves	1 large bud	30	301

Asparagus

Fresh	2/3 cup	1	183
Canned	6 spears	271	191

Beans, baked	5/8 cup	2	704

Beans, green

Fresh	1 cup	5	189
Canned	1 cup	295	109

Beans, lima

Fresh	5/8 cup	1	422
Canned	½ cup	271	255
Frozen	5/8 cup	129	394

Beets

Fresh	½ cup	36	172
Canned	½ cup	96	138

Broccoli

Fresh	2/3 cup	10	267
Brussels Sprouts	6-7 medium	10	273

Cabbage

Raw, shredded	1 cup	20	233

Cooked	3/5 cup	14	163

Carrots

Raw	1 large	47	341
Cooked	2/3 cup	33	222
Canned	2/3 cup	236	120
Cauliflower	7/8 cup	9	206
Celery	1 outer, 3 inner stalks	63	170

Corn

Fresh	1 medium ear	trace	196
Canned	½ cup	196	81
Cucumber, pared	½ medium	3	80
Lettuce, iceberg	3 ½ oz.	9	264
Mushrooms (uncooked)	10 sm., 41g.	15	414

Vegetables*

Onions (uncooked)	1 medium	10	157

Peas
Fresh	2/3 cup	1	196
Canned	3/4 cup	236	96
Frozen	31/2oz.	115	135

Potatoes
Boiled (in skin)	1 medium	3	407
French Fried	10 pieces	3	427
Radishes	10 small	18	322
Sauerkraut	2/3 cup	747	140
Spinach	½ cup	45	291

Tomatoes
Raw	1 medium	4	366
Canned	1/2cup	130	217
Paste	31/2 oz.	38	888

About The Author And Resources

Rudy Silva is a natural consultant nutritionist educated in the United State in Nutrition and Physics. He is a graduate from the San Jose State University in California. He is author of 30 other e-books on natural remedies. He has authored a newsletter in natural remedies for over 4 years. He has many websites promoting special recommended products and information.

Resource page

Here are some of the other kindle e-books about natural remedies that have been written by this author. You can see the entire list at:

http://tinyurl.com/b2f7wd3

Constipation Remedies
Best Constipated Women Natural Cures

Essential Fatty Acids

Taking The Mystery Out Of Essential Fatty acids

Amazing Fish Oil Benefits Revealed

Nutrition Remedies

Fast Healing Juice Nutrition Therapy: Nutrition Tips 3

Magnesium Nutrition Revealed

Potassium Health Secrets Revealed

A Sodium Diet (What You Must Know About Sodium)

Vegetables and Vegetable Juice Cures

Stomach Remedies

Acid Reflux: Fast and Easy Cures For Acid Reflux

Asthma Treatment Cures With Remedies

How To Do Natural Colon Cleansing

Misc. Remedies

Effective Natural Hemorrhoids Treatment

Iron Deficiency Anemia

To see all of the kindle books written by this author, go to this the Authors Profile Page or this URL:

http://tinyurl.com/b2f7wd3

If you need support or want to promote any of his e-books, please contact him at rss41@yahoo.com and expect a reply within 24 hours.

Give A Review

And, don't forget to give a review for this e-book at Amazon.

It's not hard to give a review. It can be only a sentence or two. You don't have to leave a long review. A short review helps other people decide if they want to buy a book. So give a short review and give your thoughts to help other people and to help the author improve his book.

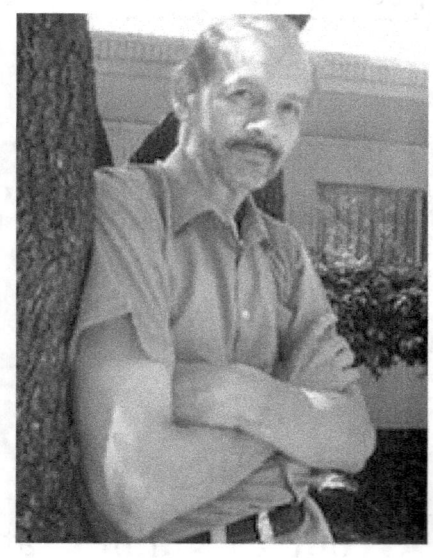

To you, for losing weight, creating better health and more happiness in your life,

Rudy S Silva